Natural Alternatives to Antibiotics

The safe remedies that work with your body to fight illness

Ray C. Wunderlich, M.D.

Keats Publishing, Inc., New Canaan, Connecticut

ABOUT THE AUTHOR

Ray C. Wunderlich, Jr. received his M.D. from Columbia University. He is board-certified by the American Academy of Pediatrics and the American College for the Advancement of Medicine and practices preventive medicine and health promotion in St. Petersburg, Florida. He is the author of many books on nutrition and health, most recently the Keats Good Health Guide, *The Natural Treatment of Carpal Tunnel Syndrome.* His other books include *Sugar and Your Health; Kids, Brains and Learning;* and *Help for New Parents and Parents-to-Be.*

Natural Alternatives to Antibiotics is not intended as medical advice. Its intent is solely informational and educational. Please consult a health professional should the need for one be indicated.

NOTE: For simplicity throughout this text the masculine pronoun is used. No gender bias is intended.

ISBN: 0-87983-684-9
Printed in the United States of America

Good Health Guides are published by
Keats Publishing, Inc.
27 Pine Street (Box 876)
New Canaan, Connecticut 06840-0876

CONTENTS

INTRODUCTION

"Vulnerability to new infections has never been greater," according to Lawrence K. Altman, M.D.[1] The apparent need for antibiotic treatment of infections has made scientists and physicians scramble to provide the medications needed to save lives and to alleviate suffering. When one considers that infections are the leading cause of death on our planet, the common use of antibiotics may seem quite appropriate. Antibiotics account for a huge percentage of all drugs prescribed by physicians. Is that desirable, or have we created a therapeutic monster that undermines our health and saps our vital state? In this text, I will identify the varied elements that comprise this issue and provide the reader a manual for coping in an antibiotic age.

The modern physician seems to possess an automatic prescription-pad reflex. He usually equates the presence of infection with the need to eradicate it by means of the most effective pharmacological agent available to him. After all, that's what a doctor does, isn't it? He acts as the arbiter in regard to the presence or absence of infection and he can recognize the "bugs" that cause infection and the drugs that knock them out. Until recently the knowledgeable matching of antibiotics to infectious diseases certainly fitted the doctor's role as an informed man of science who can alleviate human misery as quickly as possible. What is rapidly emerging now, however, is a more expanded view of the doctor and his role in society. The doctor of the near future must engage his expertise in a different way: to forestall disease and to promote vitality. In other words, more emphasis must be placed on prevention and health-building and less on disease and sickness-treating.

The present-day prescription-writing physician reflects the fact that life today has become excessively dependent upon a technologically advanced medical-pharmaceutical complex. Reliance upon one's own lifestyle to prevent and combat infections has largely flown out the window with buggy whips and isinglass curtains. Today's typical doctor prescribes more antibiotics than are necessary and frequently does not address himself to the undesirable lifestyles of his patients that foster infections in the first place. Furthermore, in rather blind devotion to the "god" of pharmacology, most doctors do not recognize or seek out more natural methods of prevention and treatment, nor do they utilize the many natural measures that are available to enhance host resistance against the sea of infectious organisms that abound in our environment.

Today, however, because of a resurgence of new infections (AIDS is just one of many) and because of rapidly developing antibiotic-resistant microbes, the scientists of the world are alarmed at the prospects for the future. The pharmacological race to develop even more synthetic antibiotics to keep ahead of drug-resistant strains is increasingly seen as misdirected, and more and more calls are being made for the curtailment of antibiotic usage, whether it be feeding antibiotics to animals to hasten their growth or feeding them to humans to counter infections. Enlightened patients, too, are objecting to the overuse of high-tech, interventional medicine and the rather casual, indiscriminate use of expensive antibiotics that some 50 percent of the time may not be required.

The message is becoming loud and clear that persons want to stay well and to avoid antibiotics whenever possible. Like a clarion call, the message is coming that legalistic, defensive medicine, fear of imperfect outcome, parental pressures to prescribe convenience and habitual practice geared to the conforming level of the community do not suffice to justify the prescription-pad reflex that triggers recurrent dependence upon antibiotics. Many persons now believe that a baby given an antibiotic for an ear infection at six months of age is three times as likely to get another ear infection within the next month as he would have been without antibiotic treatment but with natural therapies such as herbs, homeopathics, or vitamin C.

On the other hand, few if any of us would choose to live at a time before the availability of antibiotics. When one has a serious infection such as a bacterial infection of the heart valves, osteomyelitis, bacterial meningitis, blood-stream infection, contaminated wounds, or the like, antibiotics promptly used in adequate doses for a long enough time are life-saving and organ-preserving. In other, non-life-threatening circumstances, however, a host of measures is available to prevent infections or to get rid of them when they do occur by less toxic, more natural means. When properly used, these measures can sometimes completely eradicate the need for antibiotics or lessen the frequency and duration of their use. Never, however, does one wish to zealously pursue nonantibiotic measures when an infection strikes and fails to improve or grows worse. Such blind allegiance to natural therapies could result in death or serious disability. The trick is to recognize improvement or lack thereof in one's condition and to seek prompt antibiotic treatment if alternative measures fail.

To accomplish these aims it is desirable to enlist your physician's help. Some doctors will be cooperative; others will not. Let the doctor know that you wish antibiotics only for absolute necessities. Insist, for example, that sore throats be treated with antibiotics only when cultures reveal bacterial pathogens such as *group A beta-hemolytic streptococci, staphylococcus aureus,* or *hemophilus type B* organisms. Let your physician know that you are willing to be examined daily (or every six or eight to twelve hours in the case of a child) for improvement or worsening of a particular condition. Let him know that you would not hold him responsible for a bad outcome because of failure to use antibiotics at an early stage. Put that in writing, if necessary. Inform him that you are aware that he is held to a practice standard that expects him to practice medicine as his peers do, using antibiotics, and that you will not cause trouble for him. By thus cooperating and not destroying the ego strength of the physician, he may feel less threatened by your desire to rely upon alternative means that he may deem noneffective, useless, misguided, "kooky" or even dangerous. If your physician will not work with you in this way, it may be time to seek another physician.

THE CASE AGAINST ANTIBIOTICS

The primary reason for the current interest in curtailing the use of antibiotics stems from the growing numbers of antibiotic-resistant organisms isolated as the causative agents of infections. These include drug-resistant tuberculosis microbes; gonorrhea-producing organisms; staphylococcal, streptococcal and pneumococcal bacteria; enterococci; and others. Scientists agree that the over-use of antibiotics, prevalent world-wide, is the prime reason that bacteria have mutated to the resistant state. In fact, the more antibiotics are used (especially the broad-spectrum drugs that target a large number of microbes), the faster resistance develops. Remember that the sales of antibiotics have nearly doubled since the 1980s.

Furthermore, when antibiotics are kept on the shelf, susceptible strains begin to replace resistant ones again. This train of events is in many ways parallel to the march of the progress of civilization as a whole. The modern way of life provides enormous benefits to us all, but we pay for them dearly with acid rain, air pollution, highway and air accidents, litigious social climates, and environmental carcinogens. Similarly, we pay for the ready availability of antibacterial therapy with drug-resistant organisms as well as the hazards and inconvenience of drug reactions, expense, gastrointestinal disorders, super-infections with opportunistic organisms in weakened hosts, lack of healthy bowel bacteria, and yeast overgrowth. For all these reasons and the fear that killer epidemics may occur for which no antibiotic recourse may be available, an increasing cry for a more responsible use of antibiotics is being heard.

Consider that old scourge, tuberculosis. Today, new strains of the TB bacterium that are resistant to standard antibiotic treatment are occurring. The same is suspected for pertussis (whooping cough), and that poses a threat even to those who have been properly vaccinated. All sorts of new and resurgent infectious diseases currently threaten, such as Legionnaires' disease, AIDS and the Ebola virus. As *Time* magazine stated in a feature article, "The age of antibiotics is giving way to an age of anxiety about [infectious] disease. It's getting harder to enjoy a meal, make love or even take a walk in the woods without a bit of fear in the back of the mind."[2] That article goes on to quote Dr. George Curlin of the National Institute of Allergy and Infectious Diseases: "The more you use antibiotics, the more rapidly Mother Nature adapts to them." Although that landmark *Time* article did indicate that the overuse of antibiotics for people and farm animals should be curtailed, the magazine did not address the need for individuals to take charge of their health in order to forge strong defenses that infectious organisms cannot broach.

There is no question that antibiotics kill off friendly beneficial bacteria as well as pathogens. We also know that friendly bacteria exist in the intestines for the purpose of vitamin manufacture as well as local acidification and digestion. Moreover, when friendly bacteria are eradicated, the bowel usually becomes colonized with wrong bacteria that ordinarily are not found in large amounts in the bowels of healthy persons. Those unwanted guests may give off toxins that injure the liver and other organs. Long-term results such as bowel dysfunction with maldigestion, malabsorption, gas, malnutrition, polyp formation and perhaps other conditions may develop. We can gain evidence for the presence of such a toxic bowel by studying a patient's comprehensive digestive stool analysis, urinary organic acids, urine indican analysis and *Helicobacter pylori* antibodies in the blood.

Finally, antibiotics do cause allergic reactions, diarrhea, rash, upset tummies, and those ever-threatening yeast-overgrowth conditions such as thrush, vaginitis and gastro-intestinal dysfunction. Many patients become allergic to nearly all readily available antibiotics. That means that they have reached a state in which the body has told its owner: "You shall not have antibiotics." These patients are highly motivated to discover and follow any and all techniques that will allow them to live in comfort without illness and without antibiotics. Fortunately, most of the time, strict adherence to proper living, a toxin-free surround, and appropriate nutrient supplementation can assure that their health remains unchallenged.

Who are the most common victims of long-term antibiotic therapy? Probably those who have to wage battle for the rest of their lives with recurring yeast overgrowth and its consequences. The adolescent who has been treated with antibiotics over several years for acne is seen with inordinate frequency for poor health in his twenties or thirties or later, along with the many women who have taken birth control pills for many years. Stool cultures for yeast and blood yeast tests assist in diagnosis. Other gastrointestinal problems such as maldigestion, malabsorption, presence of wrong bacteria, "leaky" gut and bowel toxicity are extremely common. The patient usually presents to the physician with fatigue, itching, nose-sinus allergies, bloated abdomen, flatulence and white tongue. In females, chronic/recurrent vaginal yeast infections may be present. Some women, however, never have vaginal yeast infections. Craving for sweets or other carbohydrates such as fruits is usually present. Mental concentration and memory are often quite poor. It is true that excellent clinical results can be obtained by appropriate anti-yeast therapy. However, I suspect and find that the susceptible individual tends to have chronic/recurrent difficulties with yeast overgrowth whenever he is under stress, whenever the diet accumulates carbohydrates (especially simple sugars, refined grain products and fruits) or whenever helping nutrients are lacking.

UNDERLYING CAUSES OF INFECTION

In order to protect ourselves better from invading bacteria by strengthening the immune system, we need to understand the underlying causes of infection.

Most of us know the factors that operate to create infections. Working late at the office night after night with only a few hours sleep is one. Excessive exposure to cold or wet or damp weather may be another. Excessive amounts of "junk food" (sugar, candy, donuts, cakes, pies, cookies, etc.) are common disruptors of the body's steady state. Mental factors such as worry, loss, uncertainty or heartbreak may pull the props out from under the body's defenses. A steady barrage of indoor pollution (strong chemicals, dust, molds, inadequate ventilation) may create the conditions needed for the invasion of "body-snatching" infectious organisms. Infection (colds, flu, bronchitis, sinusitis) is just one manifestation of the body breakdown that occurs under an unrelenting barrage of physical or psychosocial demands that are not supported by optimal nourishment.

What happens under such stresses to enable the ordinarily hapless infectious organisms to turn into life-threatening aggressors? Certainly we do not know all the answers. We do know, however, that some breech in the defense systems occurs and that strong likelihood exists that nutritional deficits are involved. That conclusion stems from the concept that unremitting and sustained body stressors can create enhanced nutrient needs due to the loss of nutrients from the body or within the body.

THE IMMUNE SYSTEM

Since a strong immune system can be judged as the *sine*

qua non by which the body thwarts infection, let us examine that immune system more closely.

When a person's body is under attack by a foreign organism (bacterium, virus, fungus, etc.), a disequilibrium in body metabolism occurs that leads to an appropriate immune response. That response involves a cooperative effort from phagocytes, macrophages, antibodies and the immune warriors called lymphocytes. In that process of restoring equilibrium and containing the assault, a bevy of nutrients is required to forge the components of the containments, to sustain their efforts, and to replenish their numbers and efficiency when the battle is won. The body's resources for mounting and sustaining the attack and post-attack maintenance are not unlimited. A full complement of nutritional factors such as sleep, rest, protein, vitamins, minerals, accessory nutrients and other substances is required for the body to emerge unequivocally successful. Whenever the immune system components have been wasted in unnecessary reactions against foods (food "allergies") or against one's own tissue (autoimmune disease), then an individual may find that his defenses are insufficient to mount an effective campaign against the germ marauders. That is why chronic food allergies may create a susceptibility to chronic or recurrent infections.

Over the centuries, a rather notable controversy occurred between the proponents of germs as the cause of infectious disease and those advocating diminished host resistance as the cause. We recognize today that infectious organisms, for the most part, wait in the wings for host resistance to flag, and then they attack. Through the work of Paul Ehrlich, the existence of humoral (antibody) resistance was established, and Metchnikoff's observation led to our knowledge of cellular resistance. Today we know these arms of the immune system as the antibody and cellular components.

ACID/ALKALINE BALANCE

Most infectious organisms have a tendency to prefer sweet

and acid conditions in which to grow. It is for that reason that bacteriological laboratories utilize growth media that contain sugars of one kind or another and that have an acid pH. That observation fits with the clinical observation that persons who allow their bodies to become overly sweet or overly acid run greater risk for illness (including infections) than those whose bodies are kept non-sweet and alkaline. For this reason, an avoidance of sugars along with a diet high in alkalinizing foods (most vegetables and fruits) has generally proven to be a health-generator.

An individual can gain insight into his own acid/alkaline (pH) balance by testing his urine and saliva with standard pH test strips. Such strips can be purchased in drug stores or health food stores. One should test the saliva and urine for pH values upon awakening and midway between meals. Since the purpose of the urine is to buffer the pH of the blood, more variation will probably be encountered in the urinary pH than in that of the saliva. Nevertheless, as a general rule, a pH in urine and saliva of 6.5–7.0 is desirable. Some believe that even higher values offer a higher degree of defense against disease. The use of beneficial "friendly" bacteria on a regular basis can trigger a series of reactions in the body that insure body alkalinity on the basis of alkaline pancreatic secretions. Those friendly bacteria include *lactobacillus acidophilus* and others. Thus, the best defense against infection is a well-fed, non-sweet alkaline body with optimal bowel function i.e. a bowel movement every eight to twelve hours.

THE IMPORTANCE OF DIET AND ENVIRONMENT

Diet is a central issue in staying well and its role in infection is no exception. Here are some factors that relate to infections. A diet high in nuts and chocolate may precipitate *herpes* virus infections. Excess carbohydrates—especially sugars, fruits and juices—promote *Candida* yeast overgrowth. Milk and cheese are directly related to sinus and throat infections. A monotonous and narrow diet tends to evoke food allergies in susceptible individuals and produces malnutrition. Excess sugars paralyze the microbe-fighting white blood cells and tend to produce "candy catarrh." Specific food allergens may invoke bacterial infection in the bladder, prostate or sinuses overnight. Skewed diets disturb the body's steady state. Improper digestion and absorption of food are very common conditions that lead to subnutrition even in the face of a good diet. Subnutrition will inevitably invite infectious disease into the tissues. Diet plays an essential role in promoting or combatting infection. The advice of a knowledgeable health professional in fashioning a proper diet is highly recommended. Quality of food, biological purity of food, moderation in dietary components and variety in food choices are always prime considerations.

At the first sign of any infectious illness, one should stop all sugars and refined processed foods and begin drinking fresh vegetable juice in copious amounts. An adult might consume a pint or even a quart per day of carrot, celery, red bell pepper, beet, parsley, romaine, spinach and cabbage juice, perhaps with other vegetables added too. Children usually require lesser quantities. An apple may also be added to vegetable juice if desired. A small amount of ginger root adds zest to the mixture.

A nontoxic environment may also go far to ward off or eradicate recurrent or chronic infections, especially those of the respiratory tract. Unclean living quarters, a gas stove in the home, a residence on a busy highway, the recurring or chronic use of pesticides, paint fumes, cigarette smoke, mold-laden air conditioning ducts, the multiple chemical exposures of indoor pollution and toxic metals and chemicals in the workplace may all prove to be highly significant factors in eroding host resistance and permitting infectious organisms to gain a foothold in the body. Then, too, personal cleanliness is essential. Remember, each of us lives in a sea of infectious organisms ready to invade our tissues whenever host defenses have been compromised. In order to reduce the need for antibiotics, we must return to the mindset of pre-antibiotic days. Often, then, if one came down with an infection, a major threat to life or limb was posed.

One thought twice about going out in crowds or about getting chilled. Now, too, we know that handwashing can be most effective in curbing the spread of infectious disease. Obviously, one must cover his mouth with a handkerchief when coughing or sneezing and, of course, stay at home in the infectious stages of contagious diseases.

VITAMIN AND MINERAL DEFICIENCIES

Gradually over the last twenty years the concept of optimal nutrient supplementation has come to be recognized as a major weapon in the war on the omnipresent sea of germs that live in, on and around us. Since the availability of sophisticated laboratory tests to probe nutrient status, we have learned that nutrient needs are indeed highly individual. Moreover, nutrient deficiency is encountered in 70 to 95 percent of the population. Even those who firmly believe they are taking sufficient nutritional supplements are often surprised to find that their cells are deficient in magnesium, zinc, asparagine, glutamine, serine, vitamin B6, vitamin B1, folic acid, vitamin B12 or pantothenic acid, to name a few.

Does taking supplemental vitamins increase one's resistance to infections? Although it is possible to suppress or lower resistance by taking inappropriate nutrient supplements, in the vast majority of cases supplemental nutrients are needed in order to bolster resistance. What nutrients in what quantities and frequencies provide the most optimal defense against infections for this individual at this time? Failing that ultimate knowledge, it is surprising what can be done with the knowledge we do have. For example, 96 healthy elderly persons averaging 75 years of age were studied to assess the difference in infections that might occur by taking a daily nutritional supplement.[3] Either a low-dose multivitamin or a placebo was taken daily for one year. Those taking the nutritional supplement experienced a 52 percent reduction in infections compared to the placebo group. Moreover, five different laboratory evaluations showed improved immune system function in the group taking the nutrient mixture.

THE ROLE OF ALLERGIES

Allergies represent an immune system gone wrong. Perhaps optimal nutrition will also permit better management of the very common allergic conditions that so often predispose to infections. In fact, a large percentage of allergic patients do lose their allergies or improve when optimal nourishment via diet and supplementation is carried out. Since allergies affect the nose and sinuses so often, we find a common scenario to be: 1) Allergic exposure (dust, pollens, molds, chemicals, foods,); 2) Stuffiness and discharge, blocked sinus openings, pain and malaise; sometimes post-nasal drip, hawking, coughing and irritated eyes; 3) Bacteria invasion of the nasal and sinus tissues so the uncomfortable patient makes a trip to the doctor to attain a pain-relieving antibiotic; 4) Blessed relief! Proper allergic management may interrupt that scenario, either by minimizing the propensity for bacterial invasion, by eradicating the allergic reaction, by enhancing host defenses or by all of those means.

The causative factors in allergy are foods, inhalants and chemicals. Inhalants include a wide variety of pollens (trees, grasses, weeds), molds, dusts and dust mites and epidermoids from animal danders. Many standard allergists greatly underplay the role of food allergy as a factor in human misery. Often foods are directly responsible for precipitating infection in the throat, tonsils, sinuses, lymph glands, bladder and urethra. The most common food allergens are milk, yeast, wheat, eggs, chocolate, citrus and beans, although it must be emphasized that any food that is consumed in large quantities and with great frequency may be a culprit. For example, allergic reactions to grains are quite common because of their prevalence in our diets.

Elimination of major food allergens and decrease in frequency and quantity of ingestion of other allergic offenders provides marked improvement in those recurrent or chronic infections linked to food allergies. Allergy skin tests and blood IgE (RAST) tests are inadequate for complete evaluation of food allergies, as I will discuss later.

STRESS

The lyrics of a song from the Broadway musical *Guys and Dolls* tell us what an unhappy love affair can do to our immune system: "A person could develop a bad, bad cold."

And all too often these colds are treated with antibiotics. More and more mind-body research is validating the message of this song: that events in our lives or our perception of them can profoundly affect our resistance to disease.

To de-stress the stressed and thus to enhance the immune system, a wide variety of techniques may be effective. I prefer a good sweaty effort in the form of a 10- to 15-mile run. My wife requires an hour of deep muscle massage. My daughter needs a long visit with a close friend. Some practice *tai chi* or meditation. My son-in-law goes fly-fishing. Whatever works and is not harmful should be practiced.

Whenever the human body becomes tied up in knots, for whatever reason, resistance to infection falls, and the likelihood of microbial assault upon the body increases. A particularly interesting story is that of a gentleman named John, who, every year around Christmas, would succumb to the ravages of a flu that put him in bed for a week or two and often resulted in his taking antibiotics. John analyzed the problem. His diet, work and physical activities were no different at that time of year, but he did notice that the muscles of his neck, shoulders and back became very tight and somewhat tender several weeks before he became ill. After some twelve years of repeated illness in this manner, John sought the services of a body therapist. Commencing a few weeks before the expected date of his illness, John saw to it that deep muscle therapy (neuromuscular therapy and myofascial release) was obtained once or twice weekly on a regular basis throughout his "danger season." John and the therapist discovered that the muscles of John's body became "tied up in knots" at the advent of fall and around Christmas-time. The body therapy released the knots and the viral flu attacks never came.

Reduction or eradication of stress can be accomplished in many persons by judicious application of a wide range of body therapies.

NATURAL ALTERNATIVES TO ANTIBIOTICS

Let us now examine the nonantibiotic tools for preventing and managing infections. Specific nutrients and practices include vitamins C and A, garlic, grapefruit seed extract, honey, propolis, homeopathics, other herbs, lysine, BHT, aloe vera, glutathione, hydrogen peroxide, colloidal silver, thymus, Oolitt tongue cleansing and bacterial vaccines.

As mentioned earlier, at the first sign of illness all sugar and "junk food" must be omitted. Emphasize fresh whole foods and raw vegetable juices and eliminate dairy products.

Assure two or three bowel movements per day, using an herbal laxative such as cascara sagrada, aloe vera juice or a bulking agent such as psyllium seed. Drink at least a quart of pure water each day and obtain sufficient rest. If the infection is localized in the skin, carefully apply hot packs four times a day to the area. For sore throats, gargle every hour with warm salt water (one level teaspoon to a pint).

VITAMINS

Vitamin C
Some persons find that a large increase in vitamin C intake helps. Adults may use up to 1000 mg (1 gram) every

hour while awake. The concept of bowel tolerance is useful: take increasing amounts of vitamin C until side effects are encountered (diarrhea, gas, mouth ulcers or urinary irritation). This means your body has absorbed all the vitamin C it can use for that day. For those who have undesirable gastrointestinal effects, try the vitamin in the form of Ester-C.

We have an excellent therapeutic tool for infection in intravenous vitamin C along with other supporting nutrients. Dr. Reid Klenner championed its use in high doses for viral syndromes. I use from five to 50 grams per infusion. Before the advent of antibiotic drugs, a very dilute preparation of hydrochloric acid was used intravenously to bolster host defense. That method of treatment can be combined with intravenous vitamin C to produce a potent "cocktail" that may avoid the use of antibiotics. The very dilute hydrochloric acid is known to increase the white blood count and to stimulate the white cells to ingest and destroy foreign invaders.

Vitamin A
Vitamin A has a profoundly beneficial effect on immune resistance. When one regularly consumes a low amount of vitamin A in nutritional supplements (5000 I.U. or less), he may find that a temporary boost with vitamin A to 15,000 to 25,000 units daily turns the tide for infection control. I prefer the emulsified or water-soluble vitamin A. If there is any doubt as to the vitamin A status of the individual, a blood level of the vitamin may be obtained. Infants and children should be given lower doses. Some practitioners use much higher dosage levels, but higher doses require close medical supervision to watch for vitamin A toxicity.

B vitamins
I like to boost the B vitamins, too, by supplying additional B complex as the presence of infection increases the need for nutrients, and the water-soluble B vitamins are among the first to become in short supply. Instead of mouthing the old comment that supplemental vitamins merely give one expensive urine, I wish to make sure that one's urine has a

nice yellow color so I know the B vitamins (specifically ribo-flavin) are getting through in adequate amounts.

GARLIC

Garlic (*Allium sativum*) can be miraculous in its anti-infectious capacity. In World War I the British wounded were treated with garlic juice on sphagnum moss applied to their injuries. When antibiotics were not available in the Second World War, the Russians used garlic for battle wounds (Russian penicillin). Folk wisdom has long seen garlic as an agent of choice for intestinal parasites. Indeed it can successfully chase away the pinworms that so often thrive in the bottoms of children. With its more than 30 compounds and elements, garlic is known to possess the highest sulfur content of any vegetable. The sulfur compound *s-allyl cysteine* is one of the most potent and valuable of the many garlic constituents. Fresh garlic can be chopped or ground and taken in juice or foods. Topically it is useful in external ear infections.

Choose garlic capsules or tablets that are not sugar-coated. In strengths up to 1,000 mg per unit, one can use one to three capsules three or four times a day to attempt to nip infection in the bud. Allergies to garlic (a member of the lily family, as are onions and leeks) do occur. If one notices any worsening of congestion, rash, cough or other symptoms, the product should be discontinued. Such occurrence is very unlikely, however.

GRAPEFRUIT SEED EXTRACT

Grapefruit seed extract (GSE), in essence, is a natural broad-spectrum anti-infective. The material is non-toxic and is used to sanitize fish and poultry. It contains bioflavonoids, amino acids, fatty acids, saccharides, phenolic compounds, tocopherols, ascorbic acid and dehydro-ascorbic acid. GSE is used for gastrointestinal upsets, flus and colds, sore throats, parasites and yeast-overgrowth conditions. It is also used in cosmetics as a natural preservative and as a mold inhibitor for various foods. Some hospitals employ it to sanitize their bedding. GSE is cost-effective and may be obtained in ear drops, topical sprays, cleansers, foot powders, capsules, tablets and liquid for oral use. It is believed that GSE has no harmful effect on friendly bacteria. Other than an occasional allergy to the product, there appears to be no reason not to use the preparation for its documented inhibition of fungi, molds, bacteria, viruses and protozoa.

HONEY AND PROPOLIS

Honey has long been used for a myriad of purposes in alleviating human misery. Some success has been reported when honey is applied to nonhealing leg ulcers and bed sores. The advocacy of Dr. D.C. Jarvis, the well-known authority on folk medicine, for honey and apple cider vinegar has helped many individuals to improve digestion and gastrointestinal infection caused by *heliobacter pylori*, an organism associated with peptic ulcer, chronic gastritis, gastric cancer and perhaps other gut conditions.

Propolis, the lining of the beehive, has antibiotic properties, but is not known to be associated with the suppression of "friendly" gut bacteria as is the case with pharmaceutical antibiotics. Propolis capsules, 500 mg each, can be taken at the first sign of infectious illnesses in doses of one or two capsules three or four times a day. There is no known toxicity. A convenient non-alcoholic propolis throat spray* containing also honey, echinacea, red clover, vitamin C, clove oil and zinc citrate may be effective in minor throat infections. It has a delightful texture, smell and taste.

*Available from Golden Pride/Raleigh, 1501 Northpoint Parkway, West Palm Beach, FL 33407.

HOMEOPATHIC REMEDIES AND HERBS

Homeopathic remedies alleviate the unwanted symptoms associated with infections. Oscillococcinum, available in most health food stores, is a homeopathic preparation that is valuable to blunt the considerably unpleasant aches and pains that accompany the flu. Also, appropriate homeopathics (which have no undesirable side effects) may sustain the body's metabolism and energy while it is under assault from infectious organisms, thus enhancing the body's inherent capacities to contain and overcome the infection.

Echinacea

While homeopathic preparations use many herbs as ingredients, a great many full-strength herbs are effective infection fighters themselves. After garlic, echinacea is perhaps the most popular immune-enhancing herb. Nontoxic, used as a liquid or in capsules, echinacea can increase the phagocytic ability of the white blood cells. It has also been shown to possess an anti-inflammatory action similar to that of the nonsteroidal anti-inflammatory drug, indomethacin. I prefer to use echinacea for several days, weeks or months and then withdraw it for use again as needed.

A major component of echinacea is *inulin*, an agent that activates the alternative-complement pathway of immunity for nonspecific host defense against bacteria and viruses. Echinacea does this by increasing a substance known as *properdin*, but polysaccharide components also bind to immune cells to enhance the activity of T-cell lymphocytes with increased secretion of interferon. The end results are increased capture or ingestion of infectious organisms by immune cells, increased levels of anti-infectious neutrophil white blood cells and increased turnover of T-cell lymphocytes.

Goldenseal and other herbs

Goldenseal is often combined with echinacea as well as other herbs such as baptisia or licorice. Lomatium, Oregon grape root and St. John's wort are other useful herbs especially for viral infections, but they require nutritional supervision. The mushrooms maitake, reishi, and shitaki, as well as ganoderma and astragalus, are some of the other herbals available to boost resistance, thus tipping the scales in favor of the host, enabling him to conquer infection without antibiotics. The adaptogenic herbs such as Siberian ginseng, Asiatic ginseng and suma can also improve host resistance when it is flagging.

OTHER HELPFUL AGENTS

Lysine

The individual who successfully counters infections without antibiotics probably utilizes his immune system more appropriately than he would otherwise. That, in turn, may gear up the immune machinery so subsequent challenges can better be managed. The amino acid L-lysine possesses antiviral activity against *herpes simplex* (the agent responsible for fever blisters on the lips and mouth and also on the genitals). In adults, doses of lysine up to 1,000 mg three times a day may be required, but usually 500 mg two or three times a day suffices to suppress an outbreak. Five hundred milligrams once or twice a day may effectively prevent recurrences. Persons who consume considerable amounts of nuts, chocolate or arginine-rich amino acid supplements may need to curtail such arginine-rich input in order to do away with herpes outbreaks. Food rich in lysine include wheat germ, pork, ricotta cheese, turkey, chicken, wild game and cottage cheese. In view of the somewhat sharp taste of raw wheat germ, the fatty nature of pork, the somewhat undesirable nature of dairy products, the suspected contamination of poultry and the relative inaccessibility of wild game, one can understand how a lysine-poor diet could readily occur.

BHT

Butylated hydroxytoluene (BHT), a synthetic antioxidant that has been used as a food preservative since the 1950s, is a highly effective antioxidant, but it also is very effective in inactivating a large number of viruses, including *herpes simplex*. The usual dose is 250 mg daily, taken with some fatty food (because BHT is a fat-soluble substance). If response is sluggish, the dose can be increased to 250 mg twice daily. In general, treatment should continue for two weeks after the outbreak has resolved. In some cases a maintenance dose of 250 mg can be employed. That dose is considered quite safe. In experimental animal studies low doses have been associated with prevention of cancer and some increase in life span. In high doses, however (much, much higher doses than stated here), promotion of cancer has occurred.

Acemannan

A substance known as acemannan may have value in treating viral infections as well as in calming inflammation. Acemannan, as well as other pain-killing compounds, anti-inflammatory agents and antiseptic substances are most prevalent in the entire aloe vera leaf (gel, sap and rind) rather than in the gel alone. Suitable whole-leaf preparations that are not excessively laxative have now been developed. The material can be applied topically, gargled or swallowed. Some persons have had good results in combatting sinusitis and sore throats by using the aloe liquid as a nasal instillation. For such use I suggest professional guidance, although Acemannan is a safe product, generally without side effects. It activates immune cells to release tumor necrosis factor, gamma interferon and interleukin 1, and is known to inactivate the following viruses: herpes type 1, measles, influenza, Newcastle and human immunodeficiency type 1.

Glutathione

Concomitant with viral infections, cellular concentrations of glutathione drop sharply. Clinical experience suggests that the use of reduced glutathione on a regular basis or at the very first sign of infection may be useful to ward off viral illness. All fruits and vegetables (preferably raw) contain glutathione, but parsley and spinach are especially rich in this valuable, protective substance. At the very first sign of a cold or sore throat, one should consume copious amounts of fresh vegetable juice, with a large proportion of parsley and spinach.

Hydrogen peroxide

Under medical supervision, food-grade hydrogen peroxide (35 percent) can be used in very small doses to combat gastrointestinal *Candida* yeast overgrowth and perhaps also colonization of the gut with toxic bacteria such as *klebsiella, citrobacter, pseudomonas* or *hemolytic E coli*. Be advised that 35 percent hydrogen peroxide is a very caustic material. Intravenous hydrogen peroxide in dilute concentrations is highly effective in the treatment of the *Candida* yeast syndrome as well as the Epstein-Barr virus/chronic fatigue syndrome. When the infectious agent appears to be well entrenched and of considerable chronicity, the intravenous hydrogen peroxide (perhaps combined with vitamin C treatments as well as appropriate nutrient support) is often able to place the patient on the path to health.

Silver

Silver has long been known as an antibacterial agent. Ancient Greeks and Romans used silver containers to keep liquids fresh. American pioneers extending the frontiers to the West often added a silver dollar to milk to retard spoilage. It is an ideal food preservative at a concentration of ⅛ teaspoon per quart. Is it any accident that sterling silver or silver plate are valuable in tableware that touches food? A majority of the world's airlines today use silver water filters to produce a noncontaminated water supply. The use of silver on the skin for extensive burns has revolutionized burn care. Presently, colloidal silver in a liquid form has become available in the wake of the mounting interest in the avoidance of antibiotics. The agent appears to have activity against a wide variety of germs, bacteria, viruses and fungi (including *Candida* yeast overgrowth). Very few side effects, if any, occur with its use. The remarkable safety record makes its use for non-emergency infectious conditions particularly appealing. Some persons elect to use a small amount on a chronic basis because of the anti-inflammatory and healing effect of the metal in the colloidal form. Some take it because of the antitoxic effect that it possesses. I have seen patients who expel dead worms when treated with colloidal silver. With the recent proliferation of colloidal silver preparations, one must be aware that all preparations may not be equally effective. Advice from an experienced nutritional professional is advised.

Thymus

A host of scientific reports validates the effectiveness of thymus supplementation in improving host resistance and combatting infections. Thymic hormones and the cell products that arise from them greatly influence that arm of the immune system known as cellular immunity. Specifically, they influence the all-important T-lymphocytes (helper/inducer, suppressor, cytotoxic, natural killer cells, killer cells and macrophages). The cellular arm of the immune system is responsible for defense against chronic viruses, fungi, yeast and parasites as well as neoplasms, aging and allergenic factors. Hence, cellular immunity is a key to proper recovery from infectious conditions as well as recovery from allergies. Potent thymus supplements can often reconstitute the cellular immune system.

Thymus may be utilized along with spleen to improve host defenses and hence to diminish the need for or frequency of antibiotic use. In children and adults with recurrent respiratory disorders, allergies, chronic fatigue syndrome, repetitive herpes virus infections, or Epstein-Barr virus infection, I find that thymus supplements reduce the time needed to become well and they frequently lower the "misery index" of the patient.

Tongue cleansing

A most important measure for forestalling infection in and around the mouth is the practice of Oolitt tongue cleansing. It may sound strange, but it makes sense to ensure superior hygiene for the most neglected organ of the body, the tongue. Occupying at least one third of the oral cavity, the tongue is the largest organ of the mouth and provides a staging area for dental disease, throat and sinus infections and gastrointestinal disorders. The tongue acts as a reservoir of "seed" infectious germs (bacteria, viruses, fungi and yeasts) that give rise to harmful organisms on and around the teeth and gums. The rough structure of the tongue surface provides a large area for accumulation of unwanted debris and proliferating microorganisms. Sore throats, sinus disease, gastrointestinal conditions and periodontal disease can be diminished or eliminated when the regular habit of Oolitt tongue cleansing is carried out.

A simple analogy indicates the rationale for the routine use of the Oolitt plastic tongue scraper. If peanut butter were to be dropped on a carpet, what would you utilize first to clean it up? Obviously, one would scrape and then perhaps later brush. So too when food deposits and microorganisms collect on the tongue's "carpet surface," a plastic Oolitt tongue scraper is required. A toothbrush used on the tongue is ineffective in removing the debris that needs to be removed twice a day. Regular scraping diminishes bacteria, fungi, food particles, tooth paste, mucus and cellular debris that collects and that is implicated in the origin of tooth decay, gum disease, bad breath, sore throats, common colds, diminished taste, cough and gastrointestinal conditions.

The total bacteria count on the top of the tongue can be reduced by as much as 50 percent after only one day of tongue scraping in comparison to one week of tongue brushing to achieve the same results. For disinfection, I often suggest that the Oolitt scraper* be exposed to three percent hydrogen peroxide after use.

Lactoferrin

A potent inhibitor of microbial growth, lactoferrin is a member of the transferrin family of chemicals, substances made within the human body but now commercially available by means of recombinant gene technology.

Lactoferrin is the iron-binding protein in milk and exists as well in every human bodily secretion. It is synthesized in the white blood cells in the blood stream. The substance exerts its antimicrobial effect by sequestering iron, thus mak-

*Deep Trading Corporation, 2906 Whittington Place, Tampa, Florida 33618.

ing it unavailable for microbial growth. Part of the protective effect of mother's milk against infant gastrointestinal infections is the presence of lactoferrin in breast milk. Commercial infant formulas do not possess significant quantities of lactoferrin, and human milk contains far greater amounts than cow's milk.

Lactoferrin retards the growth of a large variety of bacteria and some yeasts. However, it also has a direct killing effect against some bacteria and an immune-regulating effect that involves chemical mediators of inflammation.

Lactoferrin also enhances the effect of antibiotics used for infection and may replace the need for some. Reduced doses of antibiotics may be permitted when lactoferrin is used along with the antibiotic. At the time of this writing, the commercial product is just becoming available through GTS Marketing in Orange, California (1–800–829–1514). Although no negative side effects are known, cautious evaluation must be carried out until further experience is gathered.

TREATING COMMON BACTERIAL INFECTIONS WITHOUT ANTIBIOTICS

RECURRENT URINARY TRACT INFECTIONS (RUTI's)

Most women pride themselves on their personal hygiene. When particular attention is paid to immaculate genital cleansing however, RUTI's as well as vaginal infections usually decrease. Immaculate genital cleansing requires careful cleansing of the area—after each voiding and after every bowel movement. The use of a non-irritating antiseptic such as Betadine solution greatly improves the results. As every woman should know, wiping is always carried out from front to back. Frequent change of underwear is also advised. Be sure that the laundry soap or detergent used is mild. No perfumes or dyes should be allowed in the genital area: that means no bubble bath, no deodorant sprays and no colored or fragrant toilet paper. Douching of the vagina with Betadine solution may also reduce urinary infections.

Just as the vagina is the contiguous neighbor of the urethra and bladder, so too is the rectum. Frequent, complete-emptying bowel movements are necessary in decreasing RUTI's. A high-fiber diet rich in whole grains, fresh fruits, and vegetable greens is essential for prompt and easy bowel function. Herbal laxatives and bulking agents such as psyllium, glucomannan, cellulose, guar, pectin or locust gum may be needed if the fibrous food doesn't do the job.

Overgrowth of *Candida* yeast must always be considered as a possible underlying factor in the woman with RUTI. The yeast may colonize the bladder or the walls of the urethral channel, thus causing irritation or urethral narrowing. One may or may not find yeast in the urine; its absence does not exclude the condition. In some cases the initial manifestation of the yeast-overgrowth disorder is urinary tract infection.

At times, either because of congenital narrowing, chronic yeast overgrowth or repeated inflammation and scarring, the urethral channel may tighten down and require repeated dilatations by a urologist. Such procedures can be helpful in interrupting the recurrent cycle of urethral and bladder infections, antibiotics, yeast overgrowth (often unrecognized by the physician) and further antibiotic treatments.

One must, of course, drink copious amounts of pure water to keep the urinary stream flowing in a full manner. Remember, the full stream carries away foreign material (including bacteria) and does away with stagnant waters that allow bacteria to multiply. Cranberries have long been used to improve the urinary system. Although many urologists scoff at the therapeutic power of cranberries, folk wisdom, as well as the clinical experience of many doctors, confirms the great value of cranberries to counter urinary infections.

Most recently, the use of cranberry for urinary tract infections has been found to be effective in a Harvard Medical School Study.[4] Seventy-eight elderly females were studied.

They drank ten ounces of cranberry juice daily or a placebo drink that was exactly like cranberry juice except that it did not contain cranberry juice. The women consuming the cranberry juice had many fewer bacteria and pus cells in their urine than those who drank the placebo.

From other studies we know that bacteria are rendered less able to stick to epithelial surfaces (such as the lining of the urinary tract) in the presence of cranberry. We know it contains hippuric acid, a natural antibiotic, but there may be other compounds as well that account for the effectiveness of cranberry. Cranberry juice is popular, but only when some kind of sweetener is added to make it palatable. The use of cranberry capsules (each taken with a large glass of water) avoids the need for sugar or fruit juice to sweeten the cranberry drink.

One could argue that home treatment of urinary infections with cranberry might relieve symptoms without actually eradicating infection. For this reason, the patient with RUTI's should be sure to have several consecutive urinary cultures done over the course of several weeks or months. If there is no bacterial growth in the urine cultures, then treatment is effective and there is little or no need to pursue further investigation in the absence of symptoms. If the urinary cultures are carefully done and turn out to be truly positive with or without symptoms, a physician specializing in urology should be consulted. A nutritionally oriented physician may be able to provide other non-antibiotic regimens to effectively manage the infection and to eradicate its cause.

One of those measures is the use of acidophilus or lactobacillus, the "friendly bacteria" to compete with or to inhibit disease-causing bacteria. To test that concept in regard to RUTI's, Reid et al. studied 41 women who had acute urinary-tract infections.[5] The women were treated with an appropriate antibiotic. Commencing on the last day of antibiotic treatment, the women were given an intravaginal suppository of lactobacillus or a placebo containing skim milk powder. Urinary infections recurred in 47 percent of the women who received the placebo, whereas only 21 percent of the lactobacillus group became reinfected. One must conclude either that skim milk in the vagina promotes reinfection of the urinary tract, that lactobacilli retard reinfection, or both.

For many years I have had women use plain yogurt vaginal douches to aid in the suppression of both vaginal and urinary-tract infections. It usually works. Commonly also, the wise physician counsels the woman to take a plentiful supply of lactobacillus by mouth in addition to local use in the vagina (and sometimes in the rectum).

Since we know that the majority of urinary infections is caused by the *E. coli* organism, we must not forget that vitamin C would also be of use. Alan Gaby, M.D. has shown that vitamin C in doses of 1000 mg four times a day helps to suppress the growth of *E. coli*.[6] In some cases, specific herbal regimens may successfully interdict urinary infection. Bearberry, pipsissewa and Oregon grape root are particularly useful. Chinese herbal combinations may work. Finally, if antibiotics must be used, any and all of the previous measures may be employed at the same time and for at least two weeks after the infection has cleared to discourage recurrence.

Women with RUTI's must also address the issue of sexual activity. Whenever one is seriously attempting to eradicate urinary infections, a period of sexual abstinence must be strongly considered. If sexual activity is to be undertaken, caution must be exercised to minimize bladder trauma as well as the introduction of foreign bacteria into the vulvar area. Careful cleansing of the vulvo-vaginal area with an antiseptic such as Betadine solution before and after the sex act may be helpful.

Remember, also, that yeast overgrowth in the urinary tract can give rise to symptoms that mimic bacterial infection (pressure over the bladder, pain in the kidney areas, inordinate frequency of urination, burning with urination, etc.). Thus an accurate medical diagnosis is essential.

Another helpful measure to diminish RUTI's is the appropriate use of natural hormone therapies. When a woman has an inadequate level of sex hormones, her bladder and urethral tissues may suffer. Not only may the sexual act be painful and traumatic, but the bladder itself may become more inviting to bacteria. Although postmenopausal women most commonly require sex hormone supplementation, the need for it is not rare in adolescence and young adulthood. Hormone replacement restores atrophic vaginal, urethral and bladder mucosa toward normal and also promotes a lower, more desirable pH of the tissue, itself an antibacterial mechanism. Estrogen, progesterone, dehydroepiandrosterone (DHEA) or testosterone may be required. The natural estrogen known as estriol is safer than conventional estrogen medications which are mostly estradiol. Estriol is believed to be an anticarcinogen, whereas estradiol possesses a mild propensity to promote cancer of the breast and uterus. Estriol can be used orally, topically applied to the skin or as an intravaginal cream. In one double-blind study, the use of estriol in the vagina lowered the incidence of urinary infection by 92 percent.[7]

SINUSITIS

Recurrent or chronic sinusitis is the nemesis of many. The condition is difficult to eradicate. Decisions not to use antibiotics in management are often heroic. Cures may be difficult to achieve, but are definitely worthwhile. Many of the previously noted measures may be called upon to attempt to avoid the succession of repeated and long-term antibiotic use that the physician must often invoke to permit the damaged mucous membranes of the nose and sinuses to properly heal. The patient must become a major participant in the decision as to whether an antibiotic is called for at any particular time. He must be able and willing to tolerate some temporary discomfort and minor symptoms in order to allow nonantibiotic measures (often slower than antibiotic therapy) to work.

The sinus cavities in the head have contiguity with veins that drain from the brain. Brain abscess, meningitis, or cavernous sinus thrombosis in the brain are rare but real potential complications of infectious sinusitis. For that reason, as well as the possibility of irremediable damage to the sinus membranes, one does not wish to permit sinus infections to persist indefinitely. As is the case with nearly all infections, when one's health is continually being undermined, when other measures are not working within a reasonable time period or when the severity of the condition dictates, antibiotics must be used.

Good communications between patient and doctor are essential. First of all, one should avoid any doctor who automatically chooses antibiotic therapy as the first treatment. The sinus sufferer needs a physician with an open mind who is willing to be a partner in deciding when the condition is getting out of hand and when the sinuses and the patient who owns the sinuses are improving.

What clues can we use to decide when sinus congestion and discharge may require antibiotic treatment? Certainly the appearance of fever and tenderness and swelling over the sinuses calls for a physician's care, especially when the clear nasal drainage changes to yellow, which often suggests a bacterial infection. Remember, however, that yellow mucus alone does not necessarily denote a superimposed bacterial infection. During a viral or allergic disorder, a late-phase reaction may bring yellow mucus with inflammatory white cells without bacterial infection. As long as there is no redness and swelling of facial tissues, no change in the individual's overall status, no definite pain or tenderness in the facial bones or teeth, and as long as one can obtain good drainage of the mucus from the nose and sinuses, then there is no urgency to presume that a bacterial infection has occurred and hence no urgency to utilize an antibiotic. If the pussy drainage does not disappear within a few weeks, or does not give signs of clearing, especially when all the following helping measures have been invoked, then other medical care is needed. Sometimes that may be antibiotics alone, but sometimes appropriate surgical procedures may also be indicated.

There is no question that the prevalence of sinus trouble is related to the problem of air pollution in our industrialized world. The huge numbers of chronic sinus patients parallel the huge numbers of environmental pollutants found in outdoor air as well as in the air that we breathe in our homes, offices and cars. Many additional factors are to blame for the epidemic of sinusitis. I shall address four: structural, allergic, toxic and nutritional.

Since the sinus cavities possess small openings into the

nose for continuity of air supply into these resonating chambers, they are vulnerable to infection when those small openings become obstructed. Structural conditions within the nose can determine whether or not those small sinus openings are obstructed. A deviated nasal septum, swollen nasal tissues, polyps within the nose or sinuses, nasal foreign bodies or pussy discharge may all be responsible for blocked sinuses, with subsequent overgrowth of bacteria in the mucous membranes of the sinus cavities as well as in the mucus of the cavities themselves.

If the obstructions are capable of being washed away, then one may avoid the need of an antibiotic. Therefore, irrigation of the nasal passages with a nonirritating solution of mild salt water may be undertaken. A rubber bulb syringe can be used. Make the solution by dissolving one-half teaspoon of salt (preferably earth salt or sea salt) in a cup of water warmed to body temperature. The douching of the nose can be carried out in a variety of ways. Some merely sniff the solution into one nostril at a time. Some irrigate the nose while holding the head over a sink or basin. Most effective is to slowly introduce the saline solution into one nostril at a time while lying on one's back with the head back and the chin pointing to the ceiling. Some prefer to lie supine and hang the head off the end of a table or bed while the nasal/sinus douche is carried out. By tipping the head to one side or the other, the fluid may be encouraged to bathe the large sinuses in the cheek areas (the maxillary sinuses). With a little practice the individual rapidly comes to know the most effective procedure for himself.

Commercial saline spray products are available at most pharmacies. For those persons who are exquisitely sensitive to chemicals, be sure to check whether the saline solution contains a preservative. If it does, that individual may prefer to make his own saline solution and to carry it in a dropper bottle, spray bottle or atomizer.

Decongestant drugs, many of which are available over the counter, are extremely helpful in opening the sinus apertures. The natural herb, ephedra, or, *Ma huang*, is found in a large variety of natural sinus preparations. Usually a number of other herbal synergists are included too. When one does not have high blood pressure, heart arrythmias or other serious medical conditions, ephedra preparations may be used. Similarly, the ephedrine derivative, pseudoephedrine, can be employed. Topical use of nasal sprays such as neosynephrine may be useful when used in low strengths (⅛ or ¼ percent). In fact, a small amount can be added to the nose/sinus douching solution. Greater strengths and long-acting topical decongestants greatly increase the likelihood of tissue damage and unwanted side effects.

Antihistamines may be helpful when congestion is caused by allergy, but rarely if ever are they useful in nonallergic congestion. At all times, of course, the individual who is being treated should use the host of nutritive, dietary, and nutritional supplement measures discussed below to reap maximal effect.

Diet and supplements can assist in opening obstructed passages even when the problem is primarily of a structural nature. Eating horseradish, strong pepper, cayenne or very warm foods may help to clear the sinuses. The bioflavonoid quercitin in doses of 500 to 600 mg twice a day in combination with body tolerance doses of vitamin C should also be used. Pantothenic acid in high doses may be helpful. I have already noted vitamin A and the other immune-enhancing herbs and homeopathics that may provide excellent help. Rather consistent decongestion of sinuses can be obtained by the exertion of steady pressure over the cheeks on both sides of the nose just below the cheekbones. Acupuncture or reflexology treatments of the feet and hands are also important tools for relief.

When structural problems prove unremitting and when they are clearly standing in the way of attaining good health, then surgery should be considered. Repair of the deviated nasal septum; removal of polyps; extirpation of foreign bodies, spurs and enlarged nasal turbinates; creation of artificial sinus openings and other procedures may be done. Whenever possible, however, most careful evaluation of allergic, toxic and nutritional factors and their connections should have already been performed.

Common medical prescriptions today for chronically congested nose and sinus cavities are topical corticosteroid sprays. In the *Physician's Desk Reference* that describes these drugs and lists their side effects, the development of yeast overgrowth is noted. There is no question that these drugs are effective for nose and sinus congestion in many cases. Consider, however, whether their long-term use is part of the solution or part of the problem. What, for example, is the long-term effect on contiguous tissues such as the eyes? What is the long-term effect on the patient associated with possible suppression of the patient's own hypothalamic-pituitary-adrenal axis? What is the long-term effect of swallowing the residue of the corticosteroid spray on the growth of yeast in the gastrointestinal tract?

We should be aware also that the medications are commonly mixed with other chemicals, some of which are trichloromonofluoromethane, dichlorodifluoromethane, benzalkonium, and phenylethyl alcohol. Although I must admit that topical nasal corticosteroid sprays serve a purpose for effective symptom relief, I would urge the patient to consult with a professional who can evaluate and treat nutritional and allergic factors in association with a comprehensive overview of lifestyle factors in order to avoid the need for long-term use of these medications.

Some individuals who manifest chronic or recurrent nose and sinus allergies with recurrent polyps (often along with asthma or eczema, as well), possess a state of adrenal gland underfunction. These individuals need the oral administration of physiological replacement doses of hydrocortisone in order to supply the substance that their own adrenal glands do not make in adequate amounts. Those persons can usually be identified by appropriate tests of adrenal function using blood, urine and saliva. Such cases have been well-described by Dr. William Jeffreys in his landmark book: *Safe Uses of Cortisone.*[8]

Even though all that congests is not allergy, a huge percentage of chronic/recurrent sinus congestion is, indeed, allergy. Scientific deliberations will go on for many years before consensus is reached about the exact role of allergy in sinus disorders. Nevertheless, people continue to find relief when their allergic factors are identified. The trick is how to do that. Conventional allergists have all been taught that nearly all allergy has its basis in IgE (immunoglobulin

E)-mediated conditions that can be detected by scratch tests or intradermal skin testing. Accordingly they are reluctant to entertain the idea that forms of allergy exist that occur on the basis of other mechanisms, and are important. Conventional allergists end up detecting and treating IgE-based allergies and for the most part miss the detection and treatment of allergies based upon non-IgE-mediated dysfunctions. Conventional allergists believe that food allergies are relatively rare. Although some are aware of the false positives and negatives that occur with skin testing, many continue to employ that method of diagnosis. A variety of other techniques is available to uncover the very common problem of food allergies that so importantly underlies chronic/recurrent sinus congestion and that so frequently is treated with recurrent use of antibiotics.

Food elimination diets undertaken under nutritional or medical supervision are one way to pinpoint food sensitivities. The mucus-producing or congestive qualities of cow's milk and its products are rooted in folk wisdom. Whether or not a true allergy, mucus produced by milk or milk products is common. Furthermore, cow's milk is acknowledged to be the most prevalent food allergen. Certainly any person with chronic/recurrent sinus congestion that leads to infections must have a therapeutic trial of elimination of milk and milk products, whether or not an IgE-mediated allergy can be demonstrated.

Whenever we say that an individual is "toxic," we usually mean that auto-intoxication from the bowel is playing its hand. When we look at the world medical literature today, we find a growing body of science that, in effect, is corroborating the previously derided concept of bowel toxicity that is responsible for a host of body ills. High on the list of toxic effects is sinus congestion. Hence the person with chronic/recurrent sinus trouble must look to his bowels and ask himself if a toxic condition exists. The key indicators of bowel toxicity are constipation, prolonged intestinal transit time, incomplete emptying, abdominal bloating or fullness, unusual amounts of intestinal gas, foul gas, alternating constipation and diarrhea, diarrhea or poorly formed stools. In addition, anal itching, mucus or blood in the stools, coated tongue and bad breath may be tip-offs to toxic bowel. The toxicity may result primarily from incomplete digestion of foods, malabsorption or from the presence of toxic bacteria, yeast overgrowth, parasites or "leaky gut." Usually combinations of these occur along with food allergies and intolerances. The management of toxicity may be accomplished by a variety of herbal detoxifications, fasts, supplementations, colonic irrigations and liver flushes. Often persons will be greatly surprised at the degree of improvement that takes place in their health as the result of successful detoxification.

Nutritional sensitivities that cause or contribute to sinus disorders are common. In fact, one frequently encounters patients who possess structural, allergic, toxic and nutritional factors all at once. In those cases one must manage the most obvious problem first and then move on to the others. For example, in order to relieve pain and discomfort, the use of antibiotics and surgical drainage may be initially required, but one shouldn't stop there. Prompt institution of the measures that I'm describing should be quickly brought to bear lest another infection, another round of antibiotics and another surgical procedure be required. With chronic/recurrent sinusitis one must be aggressive and persistent in the use of the nonantibiotic tools in order to succeed.

Sinus sufferers, like others in our society, pay a high nutritional price for the cumulative load of well-advertised, commercially attractive, processed and refined sugar- and chemical-laden convenience foods that are so readily available and that are chronically and customarily consumed by so many. If anyone ever needed a cogent reason to tone down the intake of such foods and to replace them with more nutritionally sound foods, the misery of sinus trouble may fill the bill. Candies, cakes, cookies, pies, pastries, chips, donuts, colas, frozen yogurts and ice creams need to be avoided. Vegetables, legumes, fruits, whole grains, raw seeds and nuts, in addition to appropriate amounts of animal protein, should become the daily fare.

A nutritional evaluation of the individual is carried out by means of blood, hair, urine, stool and saliva probes as well as by history and physical examination. Often a series of intravenous treatments with nutrients, vitamin C and perhaps hydrogen peroxide will be needed. At all times care must be taken to find the individual's specific nutrient needs. Oral treatments using safe but effective doses of pure nutrient supplements (vitamins, minerals, amino acids, etc.) are nearly always required.

Two other treatment modalities may be called upon to break the back of chronic or repetitive sinus congestion and the endless repetitive cycles of antibiotics and decongestants with or without antihistamines. These measures are air filtration and gamma globulin injections.

No one can argue against pure air. The only question is how best to get it. Start by having the air-conditioning ducts cleaned out. Special filters can be used. They can be electrostatic filters, HEPA filters, carbon filters or fine-mesh mechanical filters. The filters can be arranged to service the entire house or building or they can be limited to one room.

I have emphasized that air pollution is a background factor in the production of chronic/recurrent sinusitis. Certainly no action is more important for the sinus sufferer than the avoidance of cigarette smoke; industrial air pollution; insect sprays; odors of cleaning materials, paints, lacquers, magic markers, chemicals used in copiers, formaldehyde and rug-backing chemicals in new carpets; lawn chemicals; gas stoves and other appliances; and a large number of other environmental exposures.

Some patients need the support of the antibodies provided in gamma globulin. Gamma globulin may be given by shots into the muscles or by intravenous drip. As with all medical treatments, the potential advantages must be carefully weighed against the risk of side effects. Fortunately there are very few, if any, side effects, especially with small doses of intramuscular gamma globulin.

BRONCHITIS

Chronic/recurrent sinusitis not only entails a too-frequent use of antibiotics, but it also constitutes a leading risk factor in the development of chronic/recurrent bronchitis that in itself leads the patient/physician to utilize antibiotics as a means of avoiding pneumonia, bronchiectasis, pulmonary fibrosis or chronic obstructive respiratory disease. For all these reasons and more the individual should pay close attention to the measures presented earlier for the nonantibiotic management of sinusitis.

Space does not allow a comprehensive overview of the nonantibiotic management of chronic/recurrent bronchitis and other lower respiratory disorders. I shall mention, however, the use of the herbs coleus forskolii, fenugreek and mullein that strengthen the lungs and their bronchial tissues. To thin and loosen bronchial secretions the following may be effective: drinking copious amounts of pure water, use of glyceryl guaicolate expectorant and pulmonary inhalations of N-acetylcysteine. Your doctor may prescribe SSKI (saturated solution of potassium iodide) diluted in water or juice. As Dr. Jonathan Wright has reminded us, SSKI inhibits bacteria, viruses, molds and yeast and serves as an excellent expectorant.[9] The anti-infectious aspect of SSKI becomes more familiar when we remember that iodine is used topically on the skin for the same anti-infectious purpose. The use of SSKI can reduce the frequency and severity of bronchial infections. The substance may, however, interfere with thyroid function, produce or worsen acne and elicit allergic reactions in those hypersensitive to iodine.

EAR INFECTIONS

With childhood ear infections, the trick is to withhold the use of antibiotics whenever possible, to invoke the more natural alternative measures and thus to buy time for the body to mobilize its own defenses. One must remain ever-watchful to plunge in with the use of antibiotics if and when a spontaneous resolution of the infection is not taking place. By doing that, the unnecessary use of antibiotics is curtailed, yet a high degree of confidence can be had that serious complications will be forestalled.

Welcome indeed are the new federal guidelines drawn up by the American Academy of Pediatrics for treatment of inflammation and fluid collection in the middle ears of infants ages one to three.[10] Since antibiotics are effective in only 14 percent of children given the drugs, watchful waiting has been advised since the inflammation disappears on its own in 86 percent of cases. Some parents may desire to purchase an otoscope to better monitor the condition of their child's middle ears at home. However, the skill and art of visual inspection of the ear drums of an uncomfortable, fretting or actively screaming child is no easy task. If the parents have the cooperation of a competent teacher (their physician, hopefully), then the home ear inspections can be a valuable aid to everyone concerned.

No matter who is doing the looking, however, the first rule for the child with recurrent ear infections is to maintain wax-free ear canals. If for no other reason than for maintaining wax-free ear canals, a home otoscope may be useful. When a child is acutely ill with high fever and a painful ear or ears, the last thing he needs is to undergo the procedures of ear-syringing or manual wax removal. For the child with repetitive ear infections, weekly inspection of the ear canals should be carried out. Wax can be removed by gentle syringing with water of body temperature mixed with 3 percent hydrogen peroxide. This can be carried out in the doctor's office or perhaps at home. Although folk wisdom tells us never to put anything in one's ear smaller than an elbow, judicious use of a rubber bulb syringe inserted according to the instructions of the physician can keep the ear canals in the desirable wax-free state. The wax, of course, constitutes a formidable barrier that hinders the all-important visual inspection of the ear canals and the ear drums. Physicians who must make their judgment as to the urgency of need for antibiotics need an unobstructed view of the entire surface of the ear drums. Unfortunately, too often faced with an obstruction because of ear wax, a physician may decide to prescribe an antibiotic just in case the ears are inflamed.

All of the measures discussed in the management of chronic/repetitive sinus congestion, as well as the general measures to counter infection and to boost immune defense, can be brought into play. The presence of fluid in the middle ears alone (serous otitis media) does not usually call for the use of antibiotics. If the middle ear cavity is filled with pus, however, antibiotics may be needed. Second-hand cigarette smoke in the home is one underlying cause of children's recurrent ear infections as well as repeated sore throats or sinus disorders.

An effective home remedy for earaches is garlic crushed and mixed in warm olive oil (then strained out) and dropped into the external ears of the child with middle ear infections. Oral garlic, echinacea, goldenseal, decongestants, vitamin C and various individually prescribed homeopathic remedies may also be needed. Vitamin A is also important, used in the pulse method of intermittently high doses for a few days at a time (and always under a doctor's supervision). Attention to proper diet, bowel function and allergies must be carried out. A dust-free, particle-free bedroom may be needed along with an effective room-air filter (HEPA filter). Finally, the culprit may be *Candida* yeast, a common opportunistic overgrower whenever antibiotics have been used (and sometimes when they haven't). Valid yeast treatment can completely change the course of repeated infections, but so too can removal of an offending allergen or irritant such as milk, dust, molds, insecticides or fresh paint fumes in the environment. Remember, too, that if otherwise nutritious foods are to be taken out of a child's diet, suitable replacement or substitution must be carried out or appropriate nutrient supplements supplied.

Parents know well that middle ear infections are common painful nuisances that plague the health of infants and toddlers. Middle ear infections (otitis media) are doubly difficult because visual inspection of the ear drums may not be easy to do and because small children are not able to communicate well the nature of their illness: they cannot tell you what hurts and whether they are feeling better or not. A screaming, wiggling child, who may be in pain as the ears are examined, will not allow complete examination of the eardrums. As a result, the physician may have to render treatment advice predominantly on the basis of the history, the child's appearance and the doctor's experience. Very often in these cases, an antibiotic is prescribed.

Human nature tends to limit one's vision when one has become a specialist. Ear, nose and throat doctors, well-meaning in their zeal to help children avoid complications, conduct many well-controlled studies to demonstrate the effectiveness of antibiotic treatment, placement of ear-drainage tubes (tympanostomies) and adenoidectomy. Nevertheless, they need to know equally well the importance of preventive measures that will minimize the need for antibiotics. These preventive measures would include absolute prohibition of smoking in the home, strict dust-free precautions in the home (particularly in the child's bedroom), avoidance of unnecessary chemical exposures (paint fumes, pesticides) and aggressive programs of dietary improvement and appropriate nutrient supplementation.

ACNE

Iodine may stimulate the acne process in some individuals. Therefore a therapeutic trial of iodine elimination may be used under appropriate professional supervision. Trans-fatty acids, high-fat foods and dairy products are generally not desirable in the diet of acne patients although considerable individual variation occurs. As is the case with all people, but particularly with acne patients, excessive sweets in the diet should be curtailed. Vitamin E and selenium are helpful. Zinc is often helpful too, as is supplemental vitamin B_6. In the adolescent or adult doses of zinc from 15 to 50 mg/day may be used. Candida-yeast overgrowth, toxic bowel, liver dysfunction and thyroid, gonadal or adrenal disorders should be investigated in persistent or severe cases.

Exposure to the sun has long been noted to be helpful. Vitamin A may be needed in amounts up to 100,000 I.U. per day for up to three months, but be advised that all therapy with vitamin A must be rigorously supervised by a physician. Women of child-bearing age must use effective birth control during vitamin A treatment and for at least three months thereafter. Chromium at 200 mcg per day may be helpful. Oregon graperoot, goldenseal root or barberry have all been used with some success.

WHEN ANTIBIOTICS ARE NECESSARY

Under some circumstances the use of antibiotics is a must. Some of these situations have already been pointed out. Suffice it to say that galloping infections that threaten life, organs or limbs require antibiotic use. Moreover, they must be employed promptly, in effective doses and for sufficient duration to eradicate the infection. A wound on an extremity, for example, that gives rise to a red, hot, swollen and painful area, especially when accompanied by swollen lymph glands in the groin or armpit or red streaks (lymphangitis), must be treated promptly with drugs. Any inflammatory condition that is being treated by nonantibiotic means but is failing to respond may well require an antibiotic. Foolish persistence or zealous over-belief in the therapeutic power of the natural cure must be condemned. Streptococcal "flesh-eating" disease and clear-cut strep throat require antibiotics. Bacterial invasion of the meningeal coverings of the brain or spinal cord (meningitis) require often heroic doses of antibiotics, usually given intravenously around the clock. Orbital cellulitis, mastoiditis, bacterial endocarditis, abscesses of the brain or other body parts all generally require antibiotics. Grossly contaminated wounds, compound fractures and extensive tissue damage, as in serious automobile accidents or burns, usually require antibiotics. Because of the hazard of the development of irremediable neurological dysfunction, a strong suspicion of Lyme disease may call for the use of antibiotics early in the game before a definitive diagnosis can be reached. Another tick-borne disease, ehrlichiosis, may also call for early use of antibiotics.

ANTIBIOTICS AND DENTAL PROCEDURES

What about the prophylactic use of antibiotics with dental procedures? Those persons with heart defects such as congenitally abnormal heart valves, mitral valve prolapse or other heart disorders are usually advised by their physicians and dentists to take antibiotics for a few days at the time of dental procedures, especially with prophylactic or therapeutic cleaning of the teeth and gums by the dental hygienist. The rationale for this is that the patient may develop an infection that lodges on the defective portion of the heart and that destroys that vital tissue while seeding the rest of the body with bacterial shedding.

Although one cannot argue with the logic of that rationale, one encounters many, many persons whose lives are miserable because of chronic *Candida* yeast overgrowth associated with the repetitive use of antibiotics for routine dental cleanings. Many of my patients have opted to utilize the measures outlined in this text rather than use antibiotics. Many patients also fail to inform their dentists or physician that they are not utilizing the antibiotic prophylaxis. In that way, the physician, or dentist has exercised his legal responsibility, while the patient has exercised his own will to do that which he pleases for himself. There are some cases in which such action would indeed constitute a foolish and misguided adherence to natural principles. When the heart defect is relatively minor and the patient's resistance is strong, however, the avoidance of antibiotics may prove the better course. The individual should seek out a knowledgeable physician who is well-versed in nutritional medicine, and a full discussion of the issue, setting out "pros" and "cons," should be carried out before a decision is made.

CONCLUSION

I have emphasized the difficult situations that arise as some physicians, concerned parents and patients attempt to manage illnesses with a minimum of antibiotics while other physicians, parents and patients pay no or little heed to the issue. Both groups, however, must face the same common enemy: the enormous hidden intake of antibiotics by every one of us who consumes animal foods. Per weight, animals receive 30 times more antibiotics than people do. Antibiotic drugs, mostly penicillin and tetracyclines, are given to 80 to 90 percent of animals raised for food (mostly swine, cattle and poultry) in order to hasten their growth and thus to allow faster time to market. Human infections that formerly required first-generation antibiotics now commonly require second- and third-generation antimicrobials that indeed have more killing power for resistant strains but at the cost of greatly heightened expense and more significant adverse effects on the immune and blood-forming systems of the body. And then there are those growing numbers of bugs for which we now have no effective magic bullet.

We have lived with the modern miracles that antibiotic drugs have wrought since the 1940s. We now face what amounts to an epidemic of yeast overgrowth. We worry whether the right antibiotic will be available when we need it, for example, when we sustain contaminated wounds and fractures in wars or traumatic accidents. We stand aghast when we learn that children who have never had antibiotics now are found with antibiotic-resistant organisms colonizing their bodies.

Today increasing numbers of Americans are seeking alternative nontoxic methods of sustaining the body and preventing illness. It is hoped that you will join with others to practice the measures outlined in this text and thus enhance the likelihood of remaining antibiotic-free. Remember, the best drug for an infection is the one that never has to be used.

REFERENCES

1. Altman, Lawrence K. "Infectious Diseases on the Rebound in the U.S., a Report Says." The Doctor's World, *The New York Times* Medical Science, Tuesday, May 10, 1994, section C, p. 3.
2. Lemonick, Michael D. "The Killers All Around." *Time, the Weekly News Magazine*, Medicine, Sept. 12, 1944, pp. 62–69.
3. Chandra, R. L. "Effect of Vitamin and Trace-Element Supplementation on Immune Responses and Infection in Elderly Subjects." *Lancet*, 340: 1124–1127, 1992.
4. Avorn, Jerry, *et al.* "Reduction of Bacteriuria and Pyuria after Ingestion of Cranberry Juice." *The Journal of the American Medical Association*, 271: 10; 751–755, March 9, 1994.
5. Reid, G., *et al.* "Influence of Three-Day Antimicrobial Therapy and Lactobacillus Vaginal Suppositories on Recurrence of Urinary Tract Infections." *Clinical Therapy*, 14: 11–16, 1992.
6. Gaby, Alan R. "Preventing Infections of the Urinary Tract." *Nutrition and Healing*, 1; 5:7 December 1994.
7. Raz, R., *et al.* "A Controlled Trial of Intravaginal Estriol in Postmenopausal Women with Recurrent Urinary Tract Infections." *New England Journal of Medicine*, 329: 753–756, 1993.
8. Jeffreys, William, Mck. *Safe Uses of Cortisone.* Springfield, IL: Charles C. Thomas, 1981.
9. Wright, Jonathan V. "Natural Alternative Treatments for Chronic Bronchitis and Emphysema." *Let's Live*, January 1995, p. 74.
10. Kritz, Fran. "Otitis Approach Conservative." *Medical Tribune*, 35, No. 15 August 11, 1994, p.1.

11. Dubos, Rene. *Man, Medicine, and Environment.* New York: Fredrick A. Praeger, 1968, pp. 55–57.

BIBLIOGRAPHY

Bluestone, Charles D., M.D. "Otitis Media and Tubes: Update 1994." Grand rounds presentation, All Children's Hospital, St. Petersburg, FL, December 9, 1994.

Buckman, Robert and Sabbagh, Karl. *Magic or Medicine? An Investigation of Healing and Healers.* Toronto: Key Porter Books Ltd., 1993.

Crook, William. *The Yeast Syndrome.* Jackson, TN: Professional Books, 1983, 1984, 1985, 1986.

Fisher, Jeffrey A. *The Plague Makers; How We Are Creating Catastrophic New Epidemics—and What We Must Do to Avert Them.* New York: Simon and Schuster, 1994.

Garrett, Laurie. *The Coming Plague, Newly Emerging Diseases in a World Out of Balance.* New York: Farrar, Straus and Giroux, 1994.

Lau, Benjamin, M.D., Ph.D. *Garlic For Health.* Lotus Light Publication, 1988.

Margotta, Roberto. *The Story of Medicine.* New York: Golden Press, 1967, 1968.

Murray, Michael and Pizzorno, Joseph. *Encyclopedia of Natural Medicine.* Rocklin, CA: Prima Publishing, 1991.

Schmidt, Michael A. *Childhood Ear Infections.* Berkeley: North Atlantic Books, 1990.

Schmidt, Michael A., Smith, Lendon, H., Sehnert, Kieth W. *Beyond Antibiotics, 50 (or so) Ways to Boost Immunity and Avoid Antibiotics.* Berkeley: North Atlantic Books, 1993.

Ullman, Dana. *Homeopathic Medicine for Children and Infants.* New York: G. P. Putnam's Sons, 1992.